DATE DUE

		11-10-14	
FEB 1 5 1993			
APR 2 1993			
DEC 1 1993			
JAN 1 1994			
MAR 1 1995			
APR 16 1995			
SEP 2 6 1995			
MAR 2 0 1996			
JUN 16 2004			
JUL 1 8 2012			

In The Beginning

In The Beginning

Teaching Your Children About Sex – Ages 4 to 7

Mary Ann Mayo

Zondervan Publishing House

Grand Rapids, Michigan

A Division of HarperCollinsPublishers

If you are interested in having them come to your community for a seminar on communicating with children about sex:

DECENT DISCLOSURE:
HOW TO RAISE MORALLY RESPONSIBLE CHILDREN
IN AN IRRESPONSIBLE WORLD

Dr. and Mrs. Mayo may be contacted by writing to
Reference Point, Box 8022, Redlands, California, 92375.

In the Beginning
Copyright © 1991 by Mary Ann Mayo

Requests for information should be addressed to:
Zondervan Publishing House
1415 Lake Drive, S.E.
Grand Rapids, Michigan 49506

Library of Congress Cataloging-in-Publication Data

Mayo, Mary Ann.
    In the beginning: teaching your children about sex / by Mary Ann
    Mayo : illustrated by Miriam Wingerd.
        p.   cm.
    Summary: Simple text. Bible verses, and illustrations introduce
    the principles of sexuality.
    ISBN 0-310-53480-1 (printed caseside)
    1. Sex instruction for children. 2. Sex instruction for children
    —Religious aspects—Christianity. [1. Sex instruction for children. 2. Christian life.] I.
Wingerd, Miriam, ill.
    II. Title.
    HQ53.M415   1991
    649'.65—dc20

90–25712
CIP
AC

All Scripture quotations, unless otherwise noted, are taken from the *Holy Bible: New International Version* (North American Edition). Copyright © 1973, 1978, 1984 by the International Bible Society. Used by permission of Zondervan Bible Publishers.

Edited by Mary McCormick
Designed by Rachel Hostetter
Illustrated by Miriam Wingerd

Printed in the United States of America

91 92 93 94 95 / AK / 10 9 8 7 6 5 4 3 2 1

This edition is printed on acid-free paper and meets the American National Standards Institute Z39.48 standard.

To our children:
Becky, Malika, and Joe

A Note to Parents

This is perhaps the very first book you have used to formally teach your youngster principles of sexuality. Maybe you are a little concerned about whether you are doing the right thing. Let me assure you—you are. If **you** don't establish yourself as the person your children can come to with their concerns and questions about sex, they will pick up erroneous viewpoints from someone else—playmates or ... ???

In the Beginning is not the answer to educating your child sexually. It is a tool to make your task easier. You see, by virtue of being a parent you have taken on a job that offers no retirement! As much as you might hope one book or one talk might do it, sex education is a **daily** job. It is done best when you are sensitive to the kinds of messages that you are giving naturally, as well as when you are able to seize and act on teachable moments.

Few are comfortable with this aspect of parenting. Many books try to reduce anxiety by use of cartoon characters or likening coitus to "puzzle pieces." With this book we have deliberately not done that. We want the majesty and awesomeness of God's handiwork to be the first message children learn about sex.

Miriam Wingerd's wonderful art communicates this message in a way that transcends words. We have chosen to emphasize the *feeling* dimension rather than the technical.

There is considerable focus on the concept of two sexes. Today it is not popular to accentuate our differences. God never intended that the two sexes be the source of confusion, discrimination, and pain it has become. *Together* men and women reflect the image of God—each sex bringing to the relationship significance, worth, and valuable insights and understandings that are influenced by their maleness or femaleness.

Children are to be a part of the two-sex design. Biology is not the only consideration. Families are established because they provide the healthiest and happiest environment in which children can grow up. We don't really need to look at the research although it confirms this truth—we can look instead at our neighbors or perhaps ourselves!

The importance and worth of the family must be *taught*. Thus, children are able to see and understand that their sexuality has meaning and significance **beyond** the physical. Because it has not been taught within a values-laden format, sex education in the schools has failed to make a difference in kids' behavior. Research verifies this.

What should your goals and purposes be in sharing this book with your child?

1. Establishing yourself as the source of their sexual information.

2. Building a foundation that reinforces the concept and importance of family and the integral part that sex plays within it.

3. Introduction of one of the simplest and most basic aspects of sexuality ... reproduction.

4. Strengthening **gender** identity: "I am a **boy**; I am a **girl**."

Congratulations! You are off to a good start by accepting your responsibility. Beginning with the simplest concepts will prepare you and your child for the complex issues facing the adolescent. You can do it!

Special thanks are due Miriam Wingerd whose wonderful talent goes far beyond the artist's palette. Much prayer has gone into each picture, and more than once God has confirmed the direction of our efforts by suggestions that were of "like mind." Thanks, too, for the direction of Lela Gilbert and Mary McCormick.

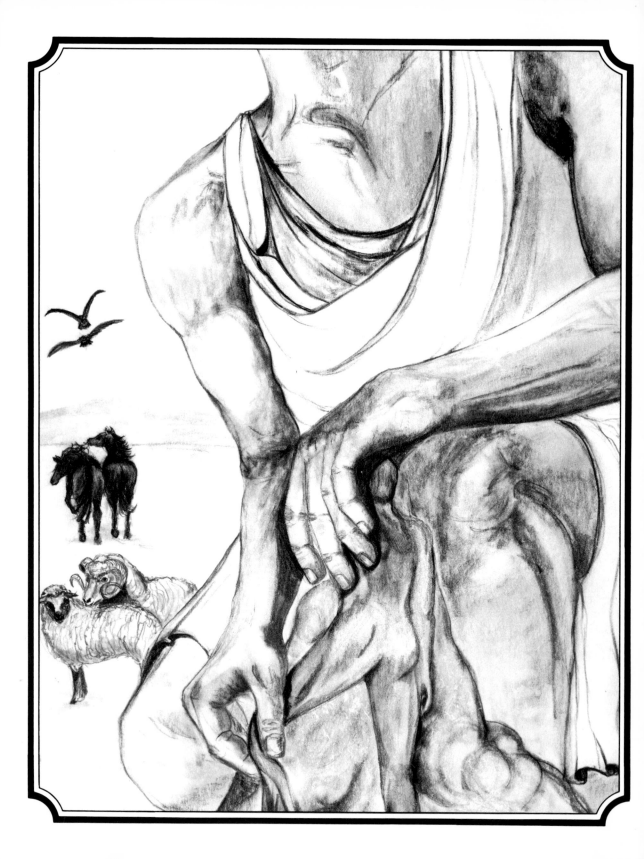

In the beginning God created the heavens and the earth. He did it all by Himself. He made it prettier, livelier, and a lot more interesting by creating plants, animals, and people, too.

He was the one who decided that giraffes would have long necks, fish would swim in the sea, and people would have little ears and walk on two legs.

Genesis 1:1 "In the beginning God created the heavens and the earth."

Genesis 1:11 Then God said, "Let the land produce vegetation: seed-bearing plants and trees on the land that bear fruit with seed in it, according to their various kinds."

Genesis 1:20 "Let the water teem with living creatures, and let birds fly above the earth across the expanse of the sky."

Genesis 1:24 And God said, "Let the land produce living creatures according to their kinds ..."

Genesis 1:26 Then God said, "Let us make man ..."

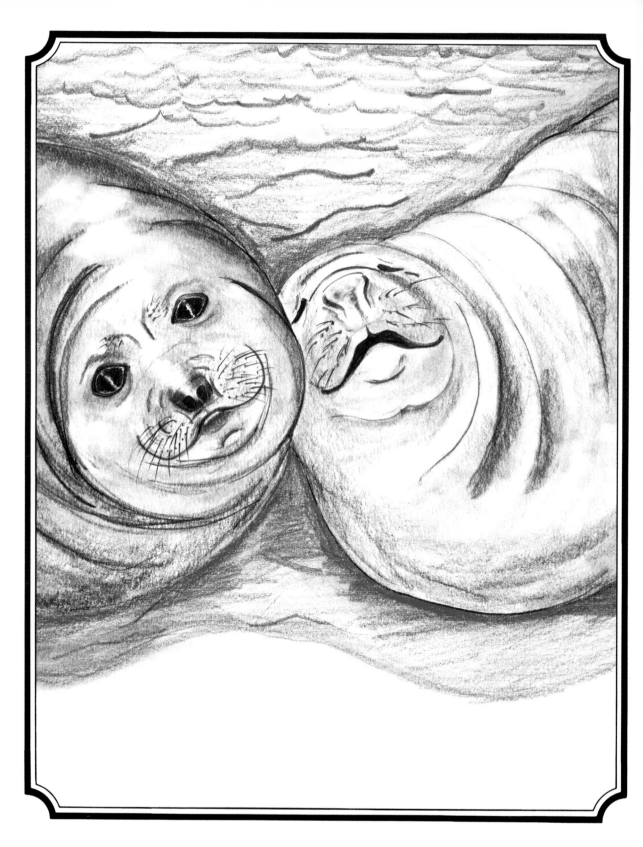

It was His idea that each plant and animal be one of two kinds—two sexes. One kind we call *male*, the other we call *female*.

Both male and female are needed before there can be any new baby plants or animals. Male and female pairs only have babies that are like themselves.

Genesis 6:19 "You are to bring into the ark two of all living creatures, male and female, to keep them alive with you."

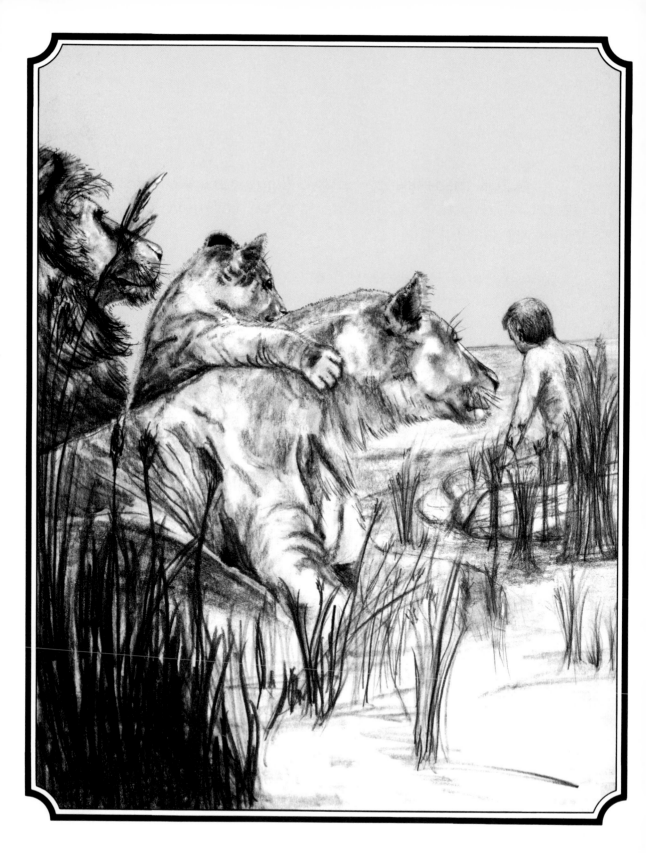

God made people in two kinds also. We call them:

boys or girls
men or women
male or female
he or she
mothers or fathers

However, He did not make the woman right away. All the animals had a mate, but the first male person, Adam, was all by himself and he was lonely. He had no one to talk to or to play with or to help him in his work. He was sad.

Genesis 2:20 "... But for Adam no suitable helper was found."

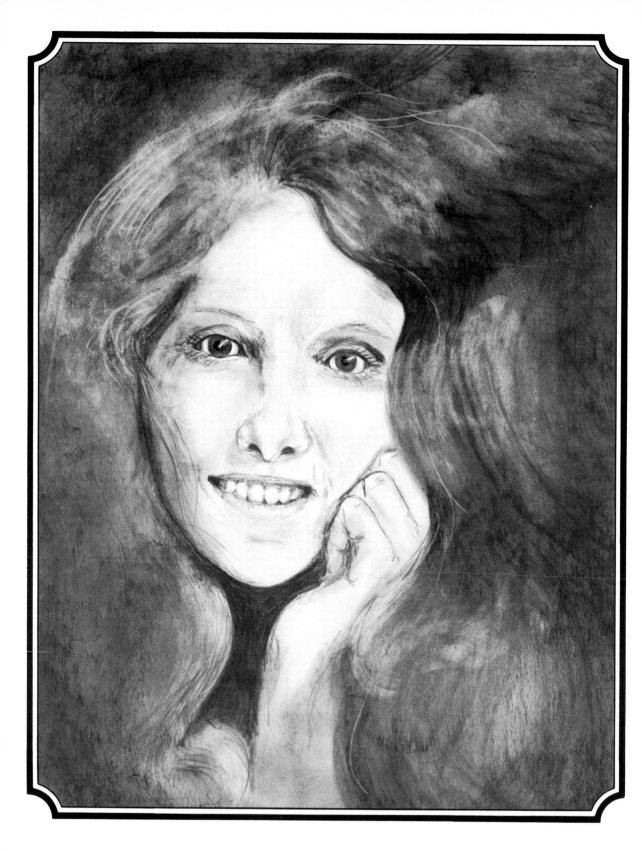

God saw that it was NOT good that Adam was alone, so He made a female person—Eve—especially for him. Eve was formed from the same material as Adam. That made them alike.

Adam said, "WOW!"

God said, "This is VERY good!"

Genesis 2:22   "Then the Lord God made a woman from the rib he had taken out of the man, and he brought her to the man."

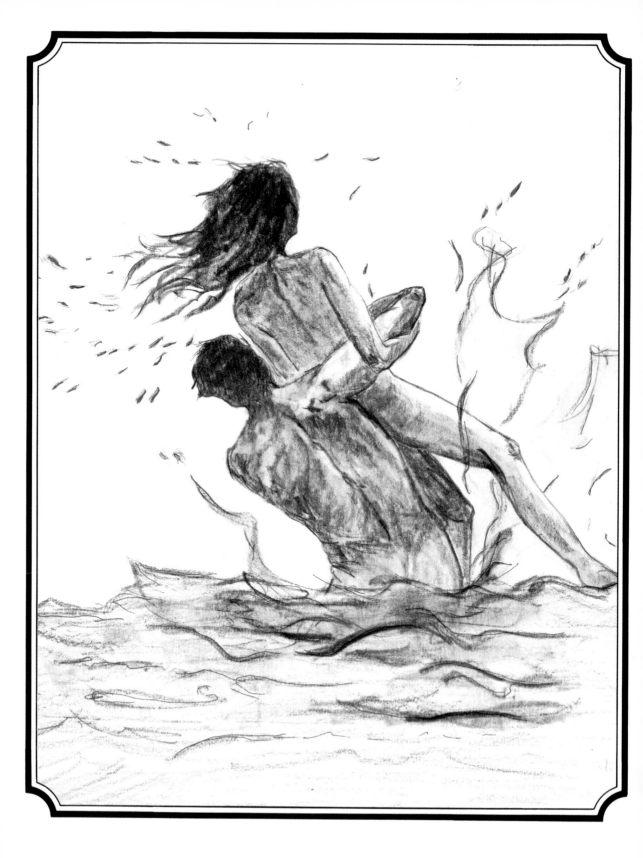

God told Adam and Eve they were specially made, for unlike the animals, they could be His friend. God also gave them an important job to do—together, they were to take care of the earth and all that was in it.

Adam wasn't lonely anymore! He and Eve were partners and shared the work, and they brought to the job their different talents.

They loved to play together, too—for they had been made perfect pals.

And because their bodies had been made in two kinds, they were able to have a baby together—something neither one could do alone!

Genesis 1:28   "Be fruitful and increase in number; fill the earth and subdue it."

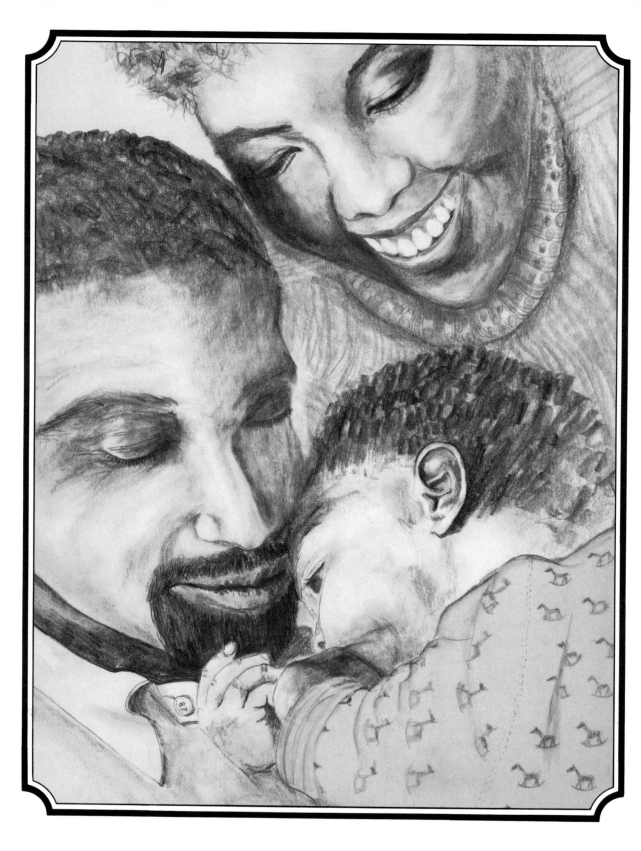

Did you know that it was God's idea that men and women would want to be together? Adam and Eve liked that idea. They were the very first *family.*

Today, men and women still want to be together. When they are grown, most leave home and start a new family of their own. A husband and wife are sometimes called a *couple.*

When you grow up, would you like to have a family of your own?

Matthew 19: 5–6
"... For this reason a man will leave his father and mother and be united to his wife, and the two will become one flesh. So they are no longer two, but one."

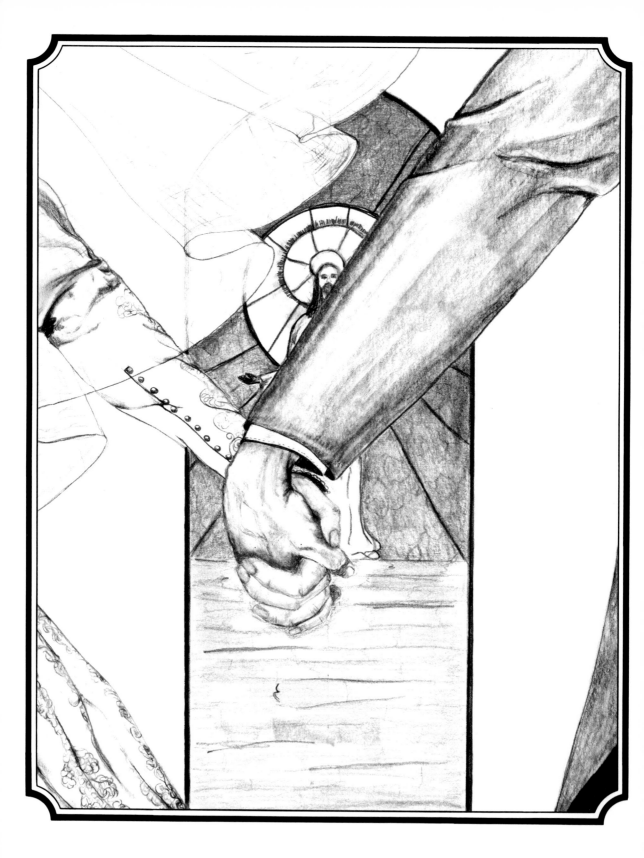

Getting married is the way couples tell everybody they have accepted God's plan to become a family.

People usually get married in a church. The special ceremony in which a couple promises to love each other forever is called a wedding. In charge is a minister who reminds everyone that being together as husband and wife is God's plan, and that *marriage* is God's desire for most men and women.

Hebrews 13:4 "Marriage should be honored by all, and the marriage bed kept pure ..."

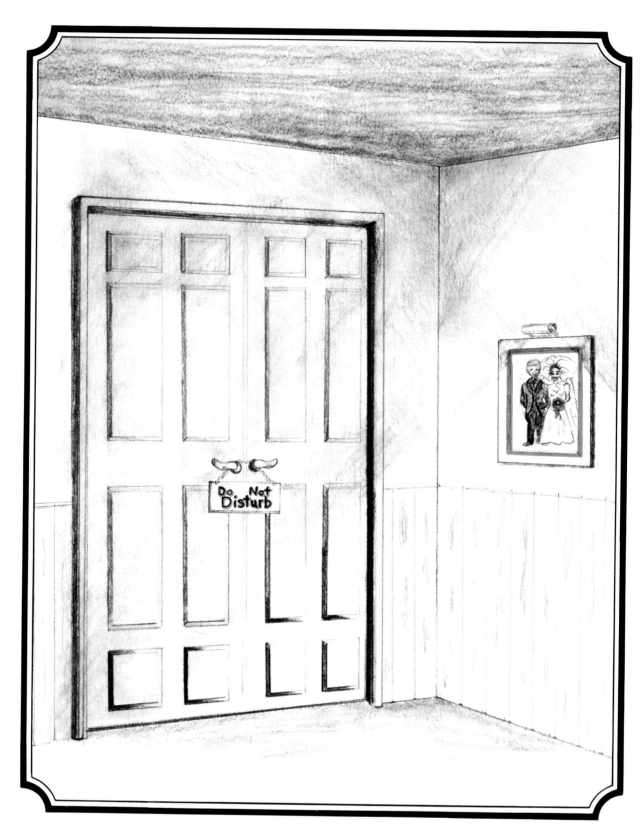

Married people like to be close in a special way.

After marriage a couple discovers a wonderful thing— even their bodies were made for each other.

Couples like to feel close and loving toward each other. It reminds them that they were made for one another.

It is during this time of special closeness that a baby can be created.

Genesis 2:25 "Now although the man and his wife were both naked, neither of them was embarrassed or ashamed" (LB).

Stages of Growth from Conception

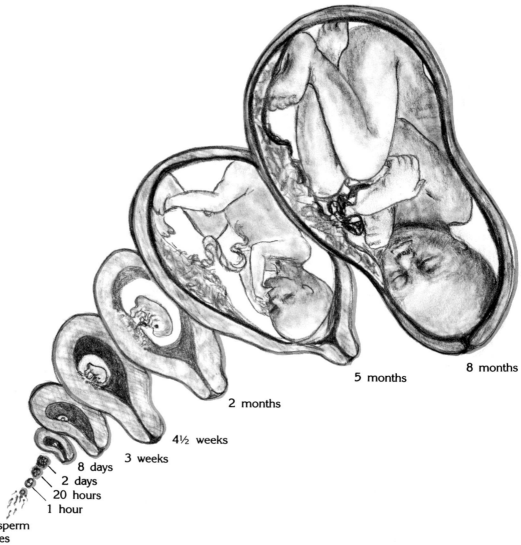

8 months

5 months

2 months

4½ weeks

3 weeks

8 days

2 days

20 hours

1 hour

One sperm
fertilizes
a ripe egg—
then conception takes place

Did you know you were born because God planned for husbands and wives to be together? He made them want to be together so each baby would be born into a family.

To begin growing, a tiny *sperm* made in your father's body and a small *egg* made in your mother's body had to join together.

God designed a man's body to make sperm and to place them inside a woman's body.

Psalm 139:13 "You made all the delicate, inner parts of my body, and knit them together in my mother's womb" (LB).

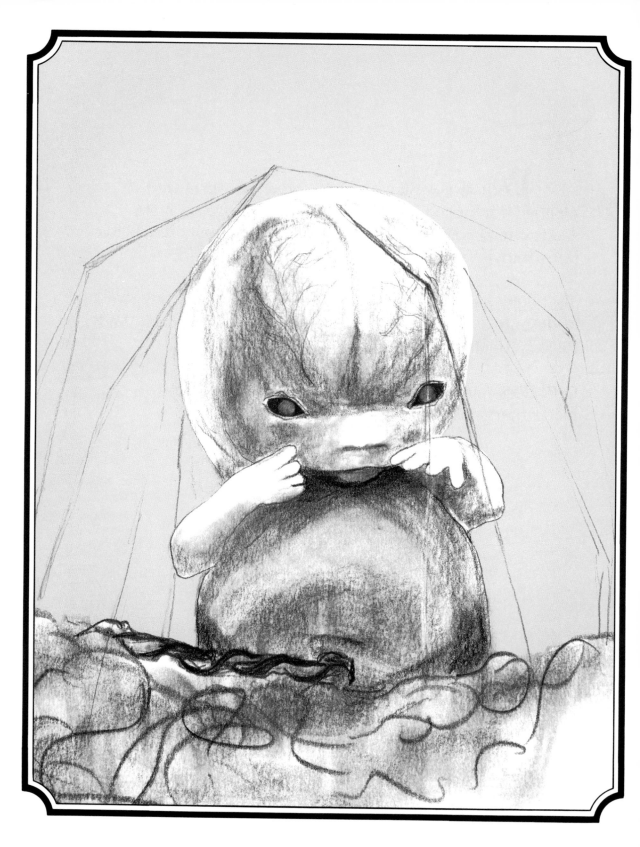

Would you like to know what happens after the sperm and egg have joined to form a baby? Babies grow and get ready to be born in a special place inside the mother's body called the *uterus* or *womb.*

The uterus (womb) is a safe place made just for babies. A baby gets its food and air from the mother through a tube (*umbilical cord*) connected to the uterus. Your belly button (*navel*) is the place where your umbilical cord was attached to your mother.

Psalm 127:3 "Behold, children are a heritage from the Lord, the fruit of the womb is a reward" (NKJV).

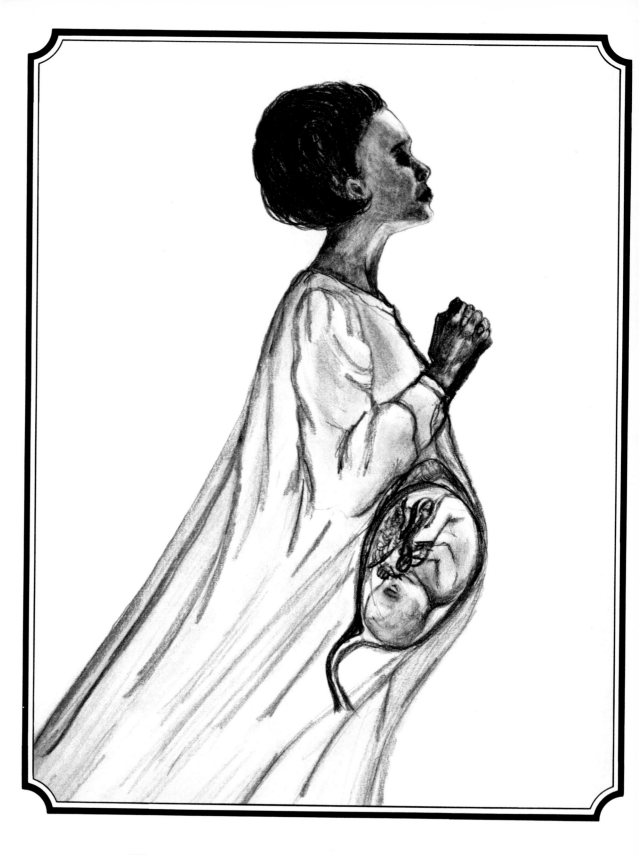

It takes nine months of growing before a baby is ready to be born and to live outside the uterus.

Psalm 139: 15–16a "You were there while I was being formed in utter seclusion. You saw me before I was born and scheduled each day of my life before I began to breathe" (LB).

At the end of nine months the strong muscles of the uterus push the baby through a tube called the birth canal (the vagina). The day that happens is the baby's BIRTH DAY.

Do you know your BIRTH DAY?

Psalm 139:16b "... All the days ordained for me were written in your book before one of them came to be."

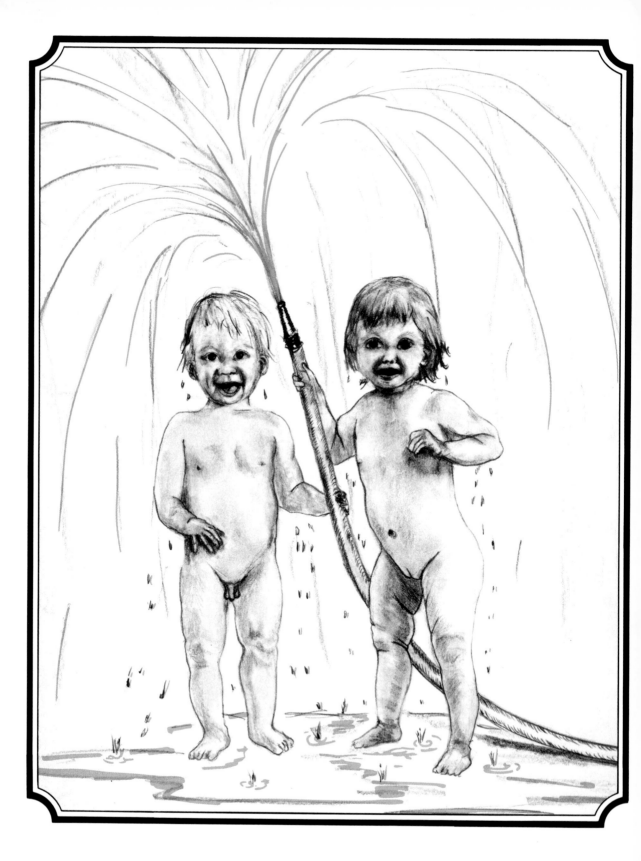

Can you guess how the doctor knows if the new baby is a boy or a girl? How do you know if God designed you to be a boy or a girl?

A boy has a *penis*. Behind the penis is a sac called the *scrotum*. This is where sperm are made when the boy grows up.

A girl has a *vulva*. Inside the vulva is the opening to the vagina.

Perhaps your family has other words for the "private parts" of the body. It is important to know their real names and purpose, too.

Genesis 1:27 "... male and female he created them."

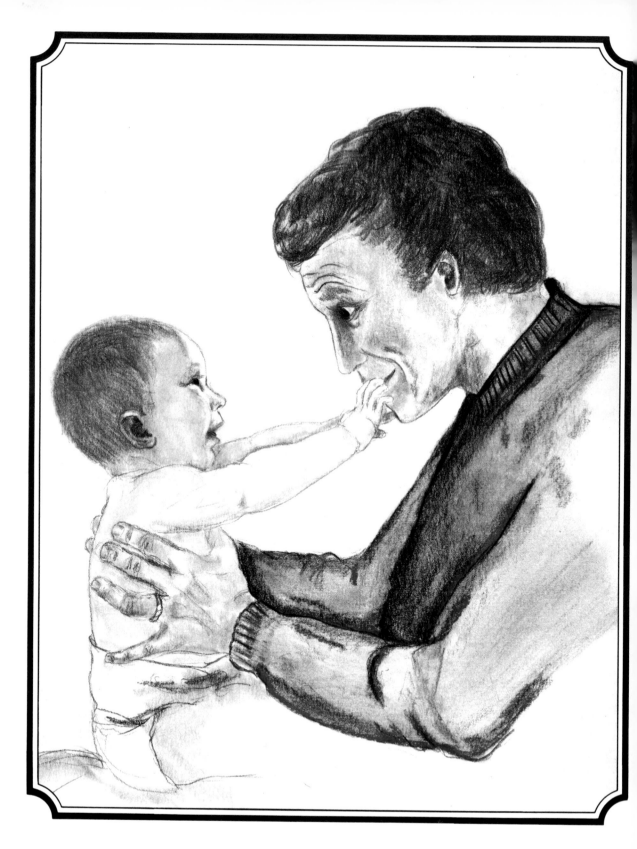

A long time must pass before a baby grows up enough to have a family of his or her own. But someday that helpless little infant will be a full-grown man or woman—and so will you.

Right now, God wants you to spend your time growing, loving, and learning about His plan for your life. Your mother and father are with you to keep you safe, to take care of you, and to teach you. Then, when the time comes, you will be ready for your very own husband or wife . . . and baby.

Jeremiah 1:4 "I knew you before you were formed within your mother's womb; before you were born I sanctified you and appointed you as my spokesperson to the world" (LB).

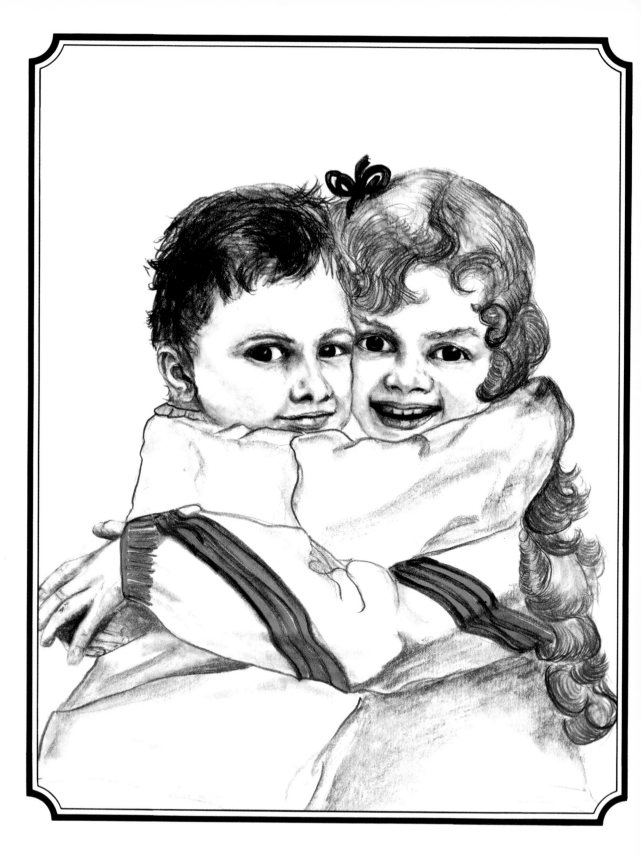

Isn't having a family a wonderful idea! God wanted each and every boy and girl to have one.

It's true that some families aren't exactly what God had in mind. But, no matter what a family is like, God still protects and loves and knows each and every boy and girl in it. And when it comes time for boys and girls to grow up and establish their own families, they have a chance to make it just as God wanted it . . . in the beginning.

And so do you!

YOU
ARE LOVED.